I0411962

# NO ONE SHOULD CARE MORE ABOUT YOUR HEALTH THAN

# YOU!

Easy insightful steps to inspire and keep you connected to all that's healthy

## Alice Cale, CHC

# How to use this book

There is continual testing involved when you're striving to be in charge of your health. It's something you probably already think about, if not every day, almost every day. This book is designed to support you on a journey that will last you a lifetime. It's meant to cheer you along as you try different things and as you actively test out what health and wellness mean to you.

Use it as a guide, kick-start, and accountability companion that will give you a push as you take the very steps needed to take control. There's a section that may introduce you to some avenues of health care that are unfamiliar. Be bold and seek out what interests you. The most important thing is for you to keep taking steps to grow and develop a plan that works for you.

Lastly, after you've tested some of the easy and simple actions, you'll be directed to a website that will keep you updated and always thinking. This site will continue to change and bring you all things healthy. Use all this information as a resource to support you being in charge!

# Acknowledgement

In 2007 I ventured out to renew a passion that I'd had my entire life. I was excited to study health and wellness and what I found was an incredible community at The Institute for Integrative Nutrition, a community of teachers, students, and ultimately fellow health coaches. To each and every one I appreciate your tenacity to carve a place for wellness professionals in the health care system.

# CONTENTS

Disclaimer: The information in this book and websites are not purposed to replace professional medical diagnosis, treatment or even advice. You should always consult a qualified healthcare professional with questions about any medical condition. The information is not a substitute for medical treatment. While all materials and links to other resources are posted in good faith, the accuracy, validity, effectiveness, completeness, or usefulness of any information herein, as with any publication, cannot be guaranteed. New England Integrative Health Counseling and it's Director accept no responsibility or liability whatsoever for the use or misuse of the information contained within or on it's website. We strongly advise that you seek professional advice as appropriate before making any health decision.

# Introduction

There's only one place to start and it's by introducing you to the person in charge of your health – That's YOU. When you look at YOU in the mirror do you see a healthy YOU looking back? Are you feeling your best every day and getting up energized and ready to meet the day?

- When it comes to your health, how well do you treat yourself?

- What's most important to you?

- Are you doing the best job you can?

Do you feel like you know what you'd like to do but can't seem to get a grasp on how to make it all come together? How you feel about yourself can make an important impact on your health and your life. On the following pages you can decide if you're ready to optimize your health. You'll be invited to take a good look at what health means to you. I'm excited to introduce you to the topics in this book. I'm sure some will be familiar and some may open new doors that may be helpful in your own personal health journey.

# Chapter One:

# Quick Start

It's funny how an unexpected occurrence can launch one into action. I decided to write this book after our family had a very unexpected health scare. It made me as a health coach take a good look at how I could step up my own game. I was content in going along thinking that my status quo was acceptable, but after recent events, I've been taking another look at what my ultimate health goals should be. For me and for everyone it doesn't make sense to expect your health to remain constant. In fact, being proactive will require assessing the changes on a regular basis, and then accomplishing a great amount of follow through.

If you feel your health is not where you'd like it, it's time to step up to the plate. Even if you feel your health is great, you need to be reassessing your goals. Strive to stay informed so you can feel confident in your decisions. If you're looking at someone else to do that job for you, reconsider that thought. Others can certainly support you but they are not able to judge how you feel and only you can truly tell what works best for you.

You'll see areas where you know you can step up your game, and to do that you'll need to take a good honest look at your current and future health goals.

While you're getting started it can be very helpful to gain the support of those around you and you may even want to bring them along. You'll be supporting them by having them become aware and become their own health advocates. As I've just learned, their health will affect your health. One of my favorite sayings is "To the world you may be one person but to one person you may be the world." I hope that statement reads true for you, and in the pages to follow, you'll find support in making your health something you stand up for. YOU are the one who needs to be in charge. It doesn't happen automatically or even with good intentions. It takes a concerted effort almost every day, but it does get easier once you've realized that you can be in control and you can take charge. You'll need to pay attention and set in motion the changes that you feel are needed. Are you ready to start? It's a lifetime commitment and hopefully a very long and productive one!

# Where to start:
# First, Question Everything

How do you feel about your health today?

What are you most happy with?

What would you most like to change?

Who do you count on first to keep you healthy ---
(Hopefully that's already you!)

What do you KNOW you should do differently?

What would your best health look like?

Why do you feel you can't accomplish your health goals?

What if you can?

Getting started will take effort, and the desire it takes to find the motivation is one of the most important things that will lead you to achieve success.

Begin by taking a new look at your goals. Some may be easy steps and some will take great resolve to achieve. It's not a fast journey but you'll find some of those goals have been coming up in your thoughts for years.

A suggestion is to look at your goals in the big picture, take on one small step at a time, and when you've written that into the pattern of your life, don't forget to do some celebrating!

It takes effort to create new habits. Your willpower may run out by the end of the day but be steadfast and set yourself up to succeed in creating that new life habit. Find ways to plan ahead. You'll have your best resolve in the early part of the day, so use it to set up ways in advance to support those afternoon downward dips. Once you've achieved writing the change into the pattern of your day, it won't continue to take that extra effort. Take a good look at how you can support creating a true change by planning and setting up ways to reach success.

Give yourself credit for every step you make. Then, without hesitation, move on to the next step. THE WAY TO START ANYTHING IS BY TAKING ACTION. When you take action, that fear and negative thoughts that have been telling you it won't work will disappear.

Be aware that sometimes all the changes you make may not be right for you. Some will work and some will not. The best thing about meeting up with a wrong decision is it will lead you to a path that's a better choice. The important thing is that you're moving forward and gaining ground on changes that will impact your health forever.

I include this next example of a conversation I often have with coaching students in hopes it demonstrates the impact that being in control of your individual goals is key. First and foremost a health coach's purpose is to support the client to take charge.

Many of the health coaching students I speak with are fearful of asking to be paid for information they've been giving away to friends and family for years. They think whatever they charge will be too much. My response to them which usually hits home is "If, with your support, your client made the changes they knew they needed or they avoided developing a chronic illness because they learned to listen to their bodies, how would you feel in 20 years when their entire lifelong health was improved? It would be priceless to them and anything you charged would not have been nearly enough."

A health coach can be one choice of support as they will encourage you to take the lead. Everyone needs support for this journey, and I hope you find it in the pages of this book.

## QUICK START

You can start to take control of your health in incredibly small steps and many times that's the best way to get started. Following may be one of the goals that is on the top of your list, maybe one that's been on your "I'll get to it" list for years. Give one a try – a simple kick-start as you read on. If one of the ideas doesn't fit for you, find a small step that does fit easily into your current lifestyle.

# IF YOU'RE
# TRYING TO CHANGE YOUR DIET

1. Be mindful

2. Take one positive step

### QUICK-START TIP:

Add more colors into your diet and look for colored veggies where the color goes all the way through!

Also take a good look at your snacking habits. Are you allowing your body to burn what you're eating? If you can make these small steps a lifestyle change, you'll start to see progress!

How about Kale & Veggies for lunch?

- Fresh kale – torn
- Quinoa or brown rice - cooked
- Garbanzo beans - drained
- Veggies you love – sliced
- Cilantro or basil
- Feta or blue cheese
- Olive oil

- You can add: free range chicken or protein of your choice.

- A favorite spicy dressing (Just a little)

- Dulse Sea Salt and pepper

(The portions of each to your taste)

Heat olive oil in pan. In a colander rinse kale & beans, adding them wet to the pan. Cover and start the kale wilting. Then add the other ingredients

until heated. Top with feta cheese

# IF YOU'RE
# TRYING TO STEP UP YOUR EXERCISE

1. Look at how you currently move your body
2. Try adding something new 7 -12 minutes each day

**QUICK-START TIP:**

Add just 5 minutes of movement at least 5 days a week

OR

If you enjoy a more intense workout try a 12 minute workout every other day. (Allow that recovery day – it's as important to restore)

How About:

An App for your phone or tablet?

My favorite:

The 7 Minute Workout by UOVO

Another tip is to try the 10,000 steps a day workout. All it takes is a pedometer and the determination to get it done.

# IF YOU'RE
# TRYING TO REDUCE STRESS IN YOUR LIFE

1.  Analyze what stress feels like to you

2.  Where does it show up in your body?

3.  What time of day does it affect you most?

## QUICK-START TIP:

Adopt a breathing exercise into your day.

Take one minute to

breathe in fully – hold – breathe out fully

Repeat for one minute.

This may help keep your blood pressure in check and is a great way to take a time out when you feel stress mounting up.


How about:

Incorporating a 5 minute breathing break into your afternoon?

# IF YOU'RE
# SLEEP DEPRIVED!

1. What is the major factor that keeps you from getting enough sleep?

**QUICK-START TIP:**

Find one busy task that keeps you up at night and make an effort to complete it earlier in the day.

Think ahead and plan to have things in place so you can wind down and relax at the end of your day.

How about:

Writing down a plan for your meals for the following day – or even the next week!

Include a shopping list!

# IF YOU'RE CONCERNED ABOUT A HEALTH ISSUE

1. Assess the concern

2. What professional do you need to consult?

3. Who might support you to make a move forward to its resolution?

## QUICK-START TIP:

Tell someone about your concern and desire to seek out a resolution.


How about:

Making it a priority!

# Chapter Two:

# Take Action

How wonderful it is that we live in a time when there are so many advances in medicine and the emerging acceptance of many alternative therapies. Yet it feels like these are two worlds on a collision path and we find ourselves stuck in the middle. You'll find an Alternative and Complementary Therapies section later and you'll find that when those two worlds meet and successfully complement each other the result can be great success.

As a health coach I hear from many people who have found wonderful success and guidance in clean living and alternative therapies. Success came only after years of suffering through trials of one medication after another only to find out that diet and lifestyle changes could make all the difference. I applaud them for their persistence to take charge and be the stewards of their own health.

Somewhere along their journey they figured out that it's their job to decide what is best for them. I hope you can find a path to be that steward of your health, hopefully never to go through such a long exhausting experience. It will start by you taking control of the things YOU KNOW you should do for yourself. But how do you take charge and heed the voice in your head, or more importantly your gut, that tells you this is right for me or this is wrong for me? It may be simpler than you think. In fact it's simple but not easy.

It's doing the things that are right for you and taking time to figure out what those things are, and then stepping up to the task of meeting your goals. Sounds good, sounds doable, but why do so many find it so hard? First you have to realize that it really is true - YOU ARE WHAT YOU EAT - and not only what you eat but what you do or how you take care of yourself. Health coaches are big on discussing Self Care. It's such an integral part of your life but many people think that taking care of others is more important than focusing on themselves. Is that you? Do you find yourself taking care of everyone before you think of your own needs? If you're a fan of Southwest flights like I am, you know they make a joke of putting that oxygen mask on yourself first, but in a real life like yours it's a must! If you'd like to step up and step into "Your Best Life" you need to take control. You need to navigate your health path and be in charge at all times.

When you've found the right answers for you, you'll then be able to add a support group or team that you can turn to for answers on how to accomplish those goals you set. This in no way takes the responsibility off of you being in charge – it's just awesome to have Peeps!

Know that if you're feeling unhealthy or you're overweight it may have nothing to do with your desire to be healthy or for that matter your willpower. It may have everything to do with your knowledge of the food that you eat. Before you take a look at your current diet it's important for you to know that if you're eating any processed foods they may have taken over how your body works. Really – the reactions that take place as you process what you eat are intense and can be altered by the slightest imbalance.

So what are you eating that you think might have something to do with altering your body's natural responses? What do you notice that changes your mood? Food can have a lot to do with anxiety and any agitations you might feel. As you get started you'll be urged to make a list of the things you suspect throw you off. That's a great place to start because your body is excellent at letting you know when it's misfiring! If your car weren't running on all cylinders you'd pay attention. It's time to treat yourself as well as you treat less important things in your life.

A great resource to learn more about why you should limit processed foods to a minimum, if any at all, is the book *The End of Overeating* by David Kessler. You'll be appalled at what is done to most processed foods. It will make clear the value of reading those labels and knowing what you're eating. It would also be a great step in taking control of your diet.

What you need to do is start adding nutritious foods that your body can use. If you're not getting enough nutrients to fuel your body – to literally keep it going - you'll find yourself grabbing anything to gain the energy you need.

What do you want? You may believe it's that nightly bowl of ice cream, but would you rather feel great when you wake up in the morning, or long for a sweet treat? Assess who's in control here! Do you want to take back your health? What's most important to you? You may think that you don't have the energy to take this on but I assure you when you do a little of this research you'll be convinced and ready to put yourself in control. Taking control back from those processed food manufacturers can be excellent motivation.

There are two additional books I'd like to mention: One is *Integrative Nutrition* by Joshua Rosenthal. In it you'll read how smart your body can be in leading you to make great selections. It's a no-nonsense approach to healthy living and you'll finish it feeling informed of what you can do to be healthier. The second book is Michael Pollan's *Food Rules*. It's the easiest read you'll find and it'll make you feel confident that you have the knowledge to make the most basic choices to achieve your goal of healthy eating. In fact, if you enjoy doing some research, seek out anything you can from Michael Pollan. Once you remove yourself from the gremlins hiding in processed foods you'll start to enjoy the true flavors of real whole foods. Things like sugar and salt will start to taste too sugary and salty and you'll wonder how they ever tasted good at all. A good quick test is to go without sugar for three days... tough... but on the 4th day many of your cravings will be subsiding and if you taste a food you used to crave it will taste different. Another great test, especially if you're a candy craver, is to substitute some over 70% cacao dark chocolate for your typical high sugar milk chocolate . Then after a time go back and taste the milk chocolate – you'll feel the sugary, lower quality, difference. The books mentioned above will give you a good idea of what to include and why when you start your journey to find what works best for you.

## Take Action

You can gain the knowledge you need to make this a reality.

Understand that it's important to Eat for Life.

Create Your Plan – a plan you can live with

Take one step at a time

It's all about nutrition

It's all about choices

It's all about what's right for you

Find a support team

Anyone you'd like to bring along for the ride?

(Remember that favorite saying of mine: "To the world you may be one person but to one person you may be the world." –Here's another one: "I love the recklessness of faith. First you leap and then you grow wings" *William Sloane Coffin.* Try leaning on both of these to get you started.)

# Chapter Three:

# Our Story

I'd like to interject here a story that I'm hoping will make you even more motivated to take care of your health and your health care. Most important is to make sure that you get involved in everything concerning your own health. So here's my story and I'm hoping it will make its mark. As I sat down to write this I wanted to go out and get a pint of Ben and Jerry's ice cream — no kidding that's for real. I know I don't do sugar well, I don't even feel good after I have sugar. You can ask anyone around me' it's not pretty. And, hey, I'm a health coach. I didn't go for Vermont's finest, I cut up a watermelon and had a bit and the urge to eat ice cream went away. A few weeks before I might have chosen the ice cream thinking it wasn't a big deal to go off track once in a while but my husband's health scare has changed all that. That experience has made me kick my thoughts that I need to be in control of my health into high gear. I'm doing that with a passion that is unstoppable because what happened was pretty life changing.

My husband is a pretty healthy guy. He has had a few very minor health concerns but in general he's on top of his game. He retired at 55 and that's stepping up your self-care if you've been in a stressful management job for 30 years. He has an Ayurvedic shake and probiotic granola just about every morning for breakfast and doesn't eat anything to excess – his motto is everything in moderation. Except sports! He plays basketball twice a week, practices Aikido twice a week and skis as much of the time in the winter as he can. (Including racing – and he wins a lot!) He recently had to visit the doctor for what was diagnosed as a minor health problem and a week later we found ourselves sitting in front of a CT scan room at our local hospital with our gastroenterologist and a surgeon we'd never met. (At that time little did we know he would become so important to us.) I can tell you I'm pretty particular about doctor selections. I've done quite a lot of research and I do take very seriously that everyone in our family should be in control of their own health. You should always feel secure that your health decisions are being decided by you. That particular day both of us felt pretty shaken as the doctors told us he had a massive infection in his pelvis, using the description that it was a 9.5 out of 10 dangerous. It was even more of a concern because blood work had shown the infection was systemic and his systems were slowly shutting down.

I'm going to digress here and tell you that all of your planning, all of your healthy eating, and all of the alternative therapies you know so well fail when you're faced with some situations, one being out of control infection. This is where modern medicine steps up to the plate and you'd better be prepared to find a way to integrate it immediately into your health plan. It's got to be a no-holds-barred resolution. You need to be prepared to put your best foot forward and make the decisions that are right for you and your family. I hear you saying "Aha – now you're making decisions for your family." That's right, I want you to be the steward of your own health but in an emergency situation it's an important component to have support and someone looking out for you. Someone needs to be your ears and take note of everything that's important. That's the support team on the sidelines I mentioned.

So there we were from what seemed perfect health to a CT scan and blood work to a 9.5 out of 10 dangerous infection. What was going through my head was "Is this the best place for him to be?" When I asked that question both doctors' response was that if we were not confident they would refer us to another hospital right away. They added that we could go to either of two centers, each 2-3 hours away. BUT they also said "If you choose to do that you must leave right now."

For my husband there was no choice. He was in surgery within an hour from leaving the CT scan room.

While we're at this point I want to take a minute to talk about pain tolerance. It played a big part in his situation getting out of hand. In his case he has an exceptionally high tolerance for pain. The doctors said that almost anyone else would have been in the office in acute pain three weeks prior to his seeing a need. They said it's a gift but can be a curse if you're in a situation where your body is trying to tell you you're in trouble.

If you know your pain tolerance is high, you need to take note of small changes in your body. On the other hand, if your tolerance is low you need to take more time to assess what's going on. I've always admired that high tolerance for pain until now. I admired it because I can have a relatively low-level pain and feel greatly affected by it. (My husband's entire body was being affected and he kept going, thinking he had a minor problem.)

If you do have a low tolerance to pain, feeling even small pain intensely, try to calm and control your suggestions to yourself. Take time to quietly look at what's going on, trying your best not to escalate the problem. Can you relate? One of my awesome doctors who is an MD with an amazing knowledge of Ayurveda suggests that it's wise not to make things worse with your assessments. (And by the way, if you don't have doctors you feel are awesome, find at least one you can turn to for advice.)

My husband's illness was the catalyst that made me unstoppable and maybe over passionate about everyone taking their own health seriously – like it's a job!

# Chapter Four:

# Begin

Begin your journey with simple steps.

Pay attention to your body's cues.

When you meet a goal that feels right for you, you'll feel a calm release. Almost like an Ahhhh! It might be good food, an exercise, or the right amount of sleep.

If you feel something isn't right for you, try replacing it with another choice and see how your body reacts.

## MAKE A PLAN

There are hundreds — no, more than thousands — of GET HEALTHY PLANS that people choose from. Many of them work and many of them don't. The key is that they work for some people and for others they're a road to certain failure.

A good place to start is with the basics. Diet, exercise, sleep and stress. You'll want to consider carefully what each means to you. When you start work at putting all four of these into balance you'll be on your way. Included in each category that follows are ideas that intend to get you thinking. You may find a plan that works for you, but be careful if it feels restrictive. If that's the case, it won't stick.

Seek out what you feel you want and need to be the healthiest you. How you get there is a decision only you can make. You'll realize that this is a journey you need to be in control of. You can find assistance but it needs to be in the form of support that assists you in doing the things that feel right for you.

## Think You Can

You can do this!When you dig deeply into how you feel both physically and emotionally, you can find the answers you need to make the right choices! In the sections below you'll find questions that will get you thinking. You'll need to be resourceful to find your best answers. Your spouse, doctor or best friend may support you but ultimately only you know the answers to these questions. Indeed you may need to find support to get you motivated. Finding a community of likeminded individuals for support can be a valuable catalyst. You might turn to a coach, a friend, or a mentor, someone who will listen as you decide how to take control of your:

# DIET,

# EXERCISE,

# SLEEP

# &

# STRESS

# Diet

Diet: The definition to use is NOT: "a dictated course or plan with restrictions of types and amounts of foods to eat to lose weight." Your diet needs to be a balance of foods that you enjoy and your body finds nourishing. Time to throw away that old definition.

What do you eat now that you enjoy and you know is a healthy choice and nourishes you?

_____

_____

_____

_____

What planning could you do to include more of these foods in your diet?

What do you eat that you know you should change?

_____

_____

_____

_____

What foods can you happily add to your diet to replace these foods?

What about your approach to foods is not serving you?

_____

_____

_____

_____

Things to keep in mind:

Portion control – question whether portions are making an impact on your health. When do you eat without being mindful?

Food and mood - how do you feel when you eat a food? Take note when you're anxious or angry after eating certain foods.

Are you hungry or thirsty?

What foods make you feel good?

# A New Grocery List

Old Questionable Foods     New Replacements

| Old Questionable Foods | New Replacements |
|---|---|
| _____ | _____ |
| _____ | _____ |
| _____ | _____ |
| _____ | _____ |
| _____ | _____ |
| _____ | _____ |
| _____ | _____ |
| _____ | _____ |
| _____ | _____ |
| _____ | _____ |

# Exercise

A better name for all that this encompasses might be *movement* but everyone looks at it as exercise so there it is. What you might consider is when do you feel most alive when you're in motion? What is enjoyable or gets you excited and moving at the same time?

What type of movement do you enjoy most?

_____

_____

_____

_____

What does your exercise look like now?

_____

_____

_____

Are you striving for more of this exercise?

Where would you like it to go?

_____

_____

_____

_____

What is an exercise or movement that you've always wanted to try?

_____

_____

_____

_____

Find movement that you enjoy and feel you can fit into your schedule.

Action steps: Start small and build

MOST IMPORTANT - If you fall back just start up again.

# Sleep

There is an overwhelming amount of research that proves sleep is a critical part of every aspect of living. Time to give sleep its due!

How much sleep do you get each night on average?

How much sleep does it take to make you feel awesome?

What does that awesome sleep feel like?

_____

_____

_____

_____

How many hours are you trying to add or take away?

You can reach your ideal amount of sleep by adjusting it in 15-minute increments. How will you change your schedule?

_____

_____

_____

_____

The following exercise can help you make changes:

I need to be in bed by:

I need to get up by:

Chart a plan:

For example, if you're going to bed at 12:00

and you need to be in bed by 11:00 to get your ideal sleep, start changing your sleep pattern by 15-minute increments at the beginning of each week.

Week One:  in bed by   11:45

Week Two:  in bed by  11:30

Week Three:  in bed by  11:15

Week Four:  in bed by    11:00


My Weekly changes:      Plot them in the 15 minute increments as above

_____

_____

_____

_____

# Stress

Even though this is the last of the big four, you may find that for you stress may be the first thing you need to address. If you're stressed about your health, all the other changes may be difficult to accomplish. Reducing stress can give you the relief you need to make improvements in all aspects of your health. Later in this book you'll find a chapter on Complementary and Alternative Therapies. There are many options there that can help you reduce your stress load.

How does stress play a part in your life?

_____

_____

_____

_____

Where do you feel that stress in your body?

What stresses are you putting on yourself?

_____

_____

_____

_____

What stresses are created by others?

What type of relaxation techniques or relaxing activities do you enjoy?

_____

_____

_____

_____

What stresses will you remove?

_____

_____

_____

_____

What stresses will remain?

_____

_____

_____

_____

How will you deal with them?

What relaxation techniques have you tested that you'd like to incorporate?

_____

_____

_____

_____

Once you've taken a good look at these four aspects of your life, you'll be on your way to seeing what's working and what needs your increased efforts. Then what? Decide the things you'd like to accomplish most. You only need to accomplish them one at a time. The point is to make changes that fit for you. You'll want to have these things be part of your everyday life, NOT a struggle or making you feel like you're depriving yourself.

# Chapter Five:

# Things to love about healthy living!

**Whole Foods —** This is so important. Take a look at the foods in your diet. Would they have been available during your grandparents' or better yet great-grandparents', lifetime? Find out if they existed before the 1950s, when manufactured foods started to become popular and the current standard American diet took form.

**Water –** Staying hydrated is probably the single most important thing you need to do. It's crucial to find a way to get your water intake up and keep it there.

**Organic -** You can't go wrong if you purchase as much of your food as you can organic. (USDA Organic is the only assured organic label.) When you purchase organic you'll avoid toxins and genetically modified foods (GMOs) that can wreak havoc on your body. Some fruits and vegetables are more important to purchase organic than others because of the types and amounts of pesticides used. The Environmental Working Group (EWG) has released an excellent guide that tells you which foods are the ones to especially avoid and others that are not impacted so greatly by conventional growing practices.

**Shop Local –** Buying fresh is something to take seriously. When you're shopping, be picky about how fresh the foods look. Make sure vegetables and fruits are firm, and feel and look freshly harvested. When you buy from a local farmer you can also find out more about the growing process. Farmers are usually glad to share so ask what crops are minimally sprayed and how quickly they're delivered to market.

**Probiotic –** Gut health is so important that it shouldn't be overlooked. Approximately 70–80% of your immune function is in your gut. Taking a probiotic, and better yet eating probiotic cultured foods, will go a long way to keeping you healthy.

**Few Ingredients –** Foods that have less than 5 main ingredients (abundant spices allowed!) is an excellent goal to strive for. That's going to just about kick out of the cupboard all the very poor quality processed foods in your diet.

**Cook** – Home cooked meals are made with love and care and it shows! Take time to sit, enjoy, converse, and especially chew your meals. Start today to plan your meals. Strive to make extra and large batches so you can take leftovers for lunch or freeze them for future meals.

# Feel-good things

**Tapping - EFT** – wonderful for relieving stress and anxiety. Tapping uses trigger points to redirect your thoughts and calm the flight or fight part of the brain.

**Meditation** – An age-old technique of calming one's thoughts. There is no right or wrong way to practice this calming technique.

**Organic coconut oil** – oil pulling – swish 1 to 2 tablespoons in your mouth every morning for 15–20 minutes.

**Lemon water** – first thing every morning squeeze one fresh lemon into your glass of water.

**Ayurveda oils** – using oils to hydrate your skin nourishes as it goes deeper to repair skin tissues.

These feel-good things are just examples of all the healthy ideas you'll find when you visit: NoOneShouldCareMoreAboutYourHealthThanYou.com

The next thing that will help you gain control is to take a look at where you can get support. Be resourceful and look into support from places that may not be familiar to you. There are many complementary and alternative therapies which range from the familiar to the very unfamiliar and some may be just what you're looking for.

# Chapter Six:

# Complementary and Alternative Therapies

The alternative and complementary therapies described in this section of the book can give you additional ideas for how you can be that in-control person regarding your health. Each practitioner can support you through their modality but you may find they also provide a great amount of support in other areas of your life.

Descriptions of each modality are provided and for some you'll find a quote from an active practitioner to give you a flavor of what to expect.

# Health Coaching

A Health Coach is someone who guides you through your health goals, supporting you to achieve a healthy balance. Will they tell you what to eat?

They'll give you choices to try and with that support you'll see what works for you.

They'll ask: What makes you happy? What fulfills you?

They'll ask what your food choices and specific goals are and how you feel about each.

Coaches cannot do the work for you and only you know exactly what needs to be done. They'll follow your lead with ideas, procedures and tips that work!

Here is a perfect definition from Joshua Rosenthal, Founder and Director of the Institute for Integrative Nutrition:

*"Health Coaches are poised to become an integral part of an emerging preventative healthcare model. By helping clients develop and progress towards their personal wellness goals, Health Coaches fill a vital void that complements and does not replace the work of*

*healthcare professionals.*

*Health coaching is now recognized by some of the most acclaimed health institutions in the country as an important tool to improve health and help lower healthcare expenditures.*

*Health Coaches help clients develop and progress towards their personal wellness goals by empowering them to take responsibility for their own health.*

*Health Coaches do not diagnose diseases; rather, Health Coaches work with generally healthy people who have made the highly personal decision of changing their lifestyle.*

*These self-motivated individuals are seeking a support system to help them progress towards their goals."*

# Cranial/Traditional Osteopathy

(This particular medical training has been a benefit to my family in ways that are impossible for me to adequately describe)

The Cranial/Traditional Osteopathy field began with the theory that there is movement between the musculoskeletal framework. A great emphasis is put on any negative movement or trauma that is placed upon the skull and even the smallest change can lead to a disorder.

A Traditional/Cranial Osteopath is seeking the road to health for their patient. The procedure is gentle and with little movement of the body.

**Why Osteopathy:**

You may visit an Osteopath for any of the ailments that you see any doctor for. Examples would be: digestive issues, ear, nose, or throat concerns, migraine headaches, respiratory allergies and asthma, orthopedic concerns such as back pain, chronic conditions, pediatric concerns and pregnancy support.

# Zero Balancing

Zero Balancing is a gentle and healing therapy.

It uses the principle of balancing energy flow among the bones and joints of the body. Zero Balancing practitioners use light pressure and traction on problem areas, coaxing your body back into harmony. The key is to construct fulcrums for the body to use to adjust and create balance.

Typically clients see a practitioner for a series of sessions and the client will be an integral part in the focus of each session. The client is fully clothed on a massage table and clients find it a powerful yet gentle healing energy. As in most healing therapies, it creates an awareness of the body and develops a trust between practitioner and client.

**WHY ZERO BALANCING:** To ease pain in the body and create fluid movement in areas that are stressed and out of balance. In addition, it can address the problems of emotional stress and insomnia. Zero Balancing can create a smooth transition to a healthier you.

*"The Zero Balancing practitioner gently engages*

*the client's physical structure (ligaments, bone, soft tissues), creating "fulcrums", (mindful) points of tension which facilitate one's energy (that which animates the structure) to re-organize and integrate with the physical body. This creates optimum functionality of the whole person, in harmony with their natural developmental processes (like setting your rudder to follow the best course, or tuning your radio to eliminate static)".*

*Cyndy Shaw*

www.equinoxhealingtherapies.com

# Reiki

Reiki is a complementary energy work that promotes healing by tapping into the natural healing properties of the body. It is a technique applied by gentle laying on of hands as the practitioner works through a guided energy life force. The hands may also be positioned just above the body. Reiki promotes relaxation and impacts one's life force, described as that energy that flows through every being. Reiki works to counteract stress in the body, which allows a flow of energy. When one has a vibrant high energy it is believed to promote wellness. Those with a minimal flow are believed to be vulnerable to illness.

A Reiki session works to balance the entire body, including the mind and spirit. The practitioner is making a transference of energy to make a positive impact on the flow within the client. The effect is often a warm relaxing sensation that allows the body to rely on its own innate healing power.

**WHY REIKI:** Someone may seek out a Reiki practitioner for physical and emotional stress reduction, to reduce areas of pain in the body, and to release emotional blocks and support general healing. The client is encouraged to relax, and as a result stress and tension can be released. Reiki is often used as a support modality for clients undergoing medical procedures and has proven very effective.

*"Reiki is a Japanese stress reduction technique which affords many clients, whether person or animal, a relaxed and peaceful feeling emotionally and physically. This form of gentle stress reduction complements other modalities, both alternative and medical."*

*Kathy Williams, Honor Wellness*

*kathy@honorwellness.com*

# Reflexology

Reflexology is a form of body work that focuses on specific points mapped out in areas of the feet. The benefits are reduction of pain, increased blood flow, and nurturing the body to repair any area where the client is feeling symptoms. The intent is to assist in healing, allowing the body to return to balance. Reflexology relaxes and relieves the body, and has both physical and emotional benefits. Some of the emotional benefits can be lessening anxiety, and stress release. The practitioner may also work on the client's hands or ears and some clients may benefit from work on all three.

**Why Reflexology:** Practitioners work with post-operative patients in their recovery. Reflexology work can be complementary to other medical care. Pregnant women find both pre and post-delivery benefits to working with a reflexologist. It is also recommended to someone looking to enhance cancer care.

# Acupuncture

Acupuncture is a modality that inserts needles into specific anatomical points. It works to correct pain messages and treats physical and emotional conditions. It's believed to be an Asian theory of medicine developed from techniques practiced in different regions. Western acupuncturists incorporate many theories from these countries. Thin, metallic needles are inserted along the skin of the body at strategic points related to the client's specific needs.

Acupuncture is a technique for balancing the flow of the body's energy. This technique can help relieve a number of ailments.

**Why Acupuncture:**

If you're suffering from a condition or pain, you may consider this alternative form of treatment.

Acupuncturists work on the entire body. Some conditions helped may be:

- Headaches

- Nausea

- Infertility

- Arthritis & fibromyalgia

- Stress

- Post pregnancy issues

- Back pain


*"There are several energetic pathways within the body that carry qi (vital energy), fluids and blood to all areas. When a pathway is blocked because of trauma or lifestyle habits, the qi and blood do not reach all areas of the body, and this creates pain or illness. This can also occur if one does not have enough vital energy. The insertion of needles in specific points along the pathways correct the imbalances and relieves the symptoms."*

*Ana Del Rosal MSAc, LAc*

*http://delrosalacupuncture.net/*

# Brennan Healing Science

The Barbara Brennan School of Healing describes Brennan Healing Science as "an enlightening system of healing that combines hands-on healing techniques with spiritual and psychological processes touching every aspect of your life." It is a system of energy work practiced by practitioners taught in the specific ways that Barbara Brennan developed. This healing science touches on all aspects of the client's life, working to improve and support all of the client's emotional and physical concerns.

Clients are guided to find deep connections within themselves so they can work to become clear on their own healing and life purpose. The practitioner will work with the client to develop their own personal aura and to develop a balance within their physical being that promotes wellness.

Barbara Brennan was a NASA scientist and studied many years to become a leading voice on energy healing. Classes are offered to expand the knowledge of this healing science, and practitioners are becoming more available.

**Why Brennan Healing Science:**

If you are looking to build upon your sense of wellbeing this can be a powerful experience. If you are dealing with chronic conditions and looking for a guiding experience, a Brennan Healing practitioner will assist you in your journey. Brennan Healing can assist if you are recovering from an injury or personal trauma.

*"Working with clients and my own personal work has given me the gift of seeing Brennan Healing Sciences completely heal a multitude of physical, emotional and spiritual disease processes."*

*Kathleen Kelly*

*Brennan Healing Science Practitioner*

*Kkelly127@myfairpoint.net*

# Lymph Drainage Treatment

Lymphatic drainage treatment is a light, gentle touch encouraging lymph flow. This technique is performed by a qualified and trained therapist. The technique can be very helpful to those with chronic inflammation and before and after surgeries. The human body depends so much on the lymphatic system and the gentle urging or massage can be of great benefit.

Lymphatic treatment can add and increase the flow of the lymph system, causing an active movement that supports the immune function. The lymph system transfers nutrients and carries away waste from the cells. Lymph drainage can support a sluggish system, actually aiding in relieving a toxic or stagnant condition.

**Why Lymph Drainage Treatment:** There are many reasons you may seek out a lymph practitioner. People who have had various surgeries that may have compromised lymph nodes or caused an edema. Any type of compromised circulation, chronic pain, or a need for toxin cleansing.

Lymphatic practitioners assess the lymph flow and map the improvement of the lymph drainage.

# The Pathwork

The Pathwork started in the late 1950s, consisting of a spiritual group that was drawn to the teachings of Eva Pierrokos. The efforts evolved into the Guided Pathwork Lectures.

Pathwork is now practiced around the world and offered in workshops, books and in group and individual studies. Pathwork practitioners guide others through their spiritual journey, a journey that leads the participant through their personal feelings, hopes and fears.

Information and names of registered Pathwork Helpers can be found through the Pathwork Helpers Association of North America (PHANA).

**Why Pathwork:** If you feel you would love to discover more about your journey in life and how to discover the very best you to move forward in the future you'll enjoy Pathwork. You may also find support in resolving old fears and moving into your best self.

*"Pathwork helps bring the unconscious into consciousness. And when we are aware of our habitual unconscious patterns we can start to change them."*

*Ellen Demers*

*http://vtwellnessdirectory.com/wellness_directory/energy-healer-ellen-demers/*

# Chapter Seven:

## The rest of our story

Here we go again!

I have a deep feeling that when something bad happens there will be good things that happen as a result. I know many people think that's a strange way to look at a negative experience but it always seems apparent and shows up for me. This thought is addressed here because just as my husband was getting back on his feet another family member wound up in the hospital with a life-threatening episode. Not good timing for the recuperating guy but certainly something that turned out to be eye opening and a learning experience. My husband was now being thrust into yet another emergency situation but this time as the support person. The experiences that unfolded were so different from the care that my husband received. This new chance to look at health choices from a different perspective has brought to light so many more things that we should be aware of in taking care of ourselves. The good thing that came out of this particular bad experience was a renewed and almost urgent passion to communicate that everyone needs to be aware and proactive of their health and access to health care. My head at that time was literally spinning with disbelief at the need for second opinions in almost every situation.

I can attest, after spending time in the hospital waiting for family members to be admitted and then again waiting an entire day for a discharge, that you don't want to miss your chance to take as much control as possible in any health-related situation. How many people have you heard say "I went along fine for 40-50 years and then look out, because everything went haywire?" What if you took your health seriously from age 20? Those who do are more likely to be in good health well past their 60s. Why would you not?

Today, almost a year after my husband's surgeries, he is still dealing with the effects from that original problem and as a result he's also evolved into being more aware. Where he would have let initial symptoms go (and toughed it out), he's being proactive, which is a much better approach for him and the doctor.

It's very interesting to take a look at the doctor's point of view. Physicians are so much better at finding a good outcome when the patient is proactive and they can begin treatment with available early interventions. Those *late to the party* consultations are hard on all involved. I imagine that all physicians would love to erase the phrase "if you'd only come in earlier" from their vocabulary. That responsibility lies with the patient.

Wouldn't you rather hear "We're so lucky that you caught this early?" At the beginning of our story it was quite the opposite situation - it was becoming almost too late. A very good friend of mine told me about a time her husband had been very sick with a cold and a fever. He was bracing through it and off to work. In his travels he happened upon a billboard with this simple phrase. "Many men die each year from stubbornness." He called and made an appointment to be seen by his doctor who said they had prevented that illness from turning into pneumonia just in time.

This also brings up another occasion when you have to step up and be your own best advocate. If you're calling your doctor's office with a concern or to make an appointment, be determined in getting your point across. Have things clear in your thoughts or, better yet, write down what you feel are your questions and concerns. Have in your mind what you feel needs to be accomplished in response to your current condition. If you feel you're not being understood or not receiving the action you'd hoped, take a breath, regroup and state that this is not what you expected from the call. Keep a cool head, which is much easier if you're initially prepared.

# Yearly Checkup

- How are my vital signs? e.g.: blood pressure, BMI

- Are there any screening tests that will be needed?

- When and how will I receive results?

- If any tests are suggested, what are they for?

- Discuss the following Diet, exercise, stress, and sleep and any concerns about them.

- What's been bugging you that you might think is insignificant. Fess up to those annoying little troubles – don't let them fester.

- Family history, concerns or risks and what you can do to prevent them.

- Go over current medications and need for continuing (including spelling of drugs that are a new prescription).

- If you have a condition, are there any new treatments that might be a better choice?

- What questions have you had in the past after you've left the office that you forgot to ask?

# Health Concern Visit

- Present a clear description of your symptoms

- What do these symptoms suggest?

- What tests will be requested?

- Who will get back to you with test results? How quickly?

- What is the course of treatment?

- What other choices are there for treatment?

- What medications, if any?  (Description, side effects and dosage information.)

- What should I expect next?

- Don't be afraid to discuss your feelings about the visit.

# Surgery and Second Opinions

- What surgery is recommended?

- What are the surgery specifics? (length of stay, anesthesia options)

- Who will perform the surgery? Where will the surgery be performed?

- How many times have you performed this surgery?

- What is the expected outcome?

- What are possible complications?

- Are there any side effects? ( from surgery or medications)

- Who would you recommend for another opinion?

- What is the cost and my insurance coverage?

- Is there anything else I need to know?

- Who can I contact for additional questions that come up?

Communications between doctors' offices and their patients are becoming better as technology links patients and allows them to become more involved in their care. Ask your health care providers if they now have links available to you for your health records and if you can direct emails to your doctor's office or the doctor directly.

How can you take responsibility for your health more seriously?

A good way to start is by doing some research. In the Alternative Therapies section of this book I described what complementary and alternative therapies can do to promote health. My family has been helped countless times by seeking out additional options. A big part of that includes discovering how your entire system can be supported to promote health or the healing process.

Functional medicine doctors also look at things in a *where does this start* and *what effect is this having on the body* approach. It's my belief that if you're able to seek out a doctor who thinks like a functional medicine physician you're on the right path to figuring out the root of your problems. There may be a functional medicine physician near you and you can find out by searching the

Institute for Functional Medicine site. If there's not one near you, ask around, because many doctors are practicing in a similar way.

Let's take a quick look at medical mistakes. It's something that is so important and yet so hard to believe.

Medical mistakes happen every day and it's noted that medical errors have been shown to be the third most common cause of death in America. The Center for Disease Control and Prevention notes that heart disease is the leading cause and cancer the second. In a study reported by the Journal of Patient Safety it was reported that up to 98,000 Americans die each year from medical errors.

What does this mean for you and your health? Another thing you need to put in that toolbox is AWARENESS. In our family we had medical mistakes that consisted of three errors in medications. I really can't say how we could have been prepared for one but the other two, as we look back, should have been obvious and the mistakes were standing up waving flags and yelling at an unbelievable volume. So what can you do to be aware that you need to check and recheck that medications and instructions are accurate? If you feel there is a red flag or something doesn't feel right, check and take action to find out the correct response. You're probably familiar with the page or sometimes pages of instructions that come attached to the prescription bag. Do you read them or do they find their way into the trash still attached to the bag? There is information there that you should know. The description of what the medication looks like is a great place to start. See if what the medication is used for applies to you. Regarding those ever-growing lists of side effects and complications, be sure to keep that paper away from the trash until you're well over any effects of the drug. In the following section you can judge how you're prepared for that immediate or emergency situation. It's something my family was fortunate to have very little experience with, but something I now see you can be prepared for.

## Good to Know

Below are some conditions that may send you or your family seeking medical help. If you have choices in your area get tuned into what the best choices for each specific situation might be. Many doctors and hospitals are known for their specialties.

- Acute trauma

- Stomach pain

- Broken bones and injury

- Throat/Respiratory infections

- Bruises/Cuts

- Back/Neck Pain

- Rashes/Infections

- Headaches

- Facial/Teeth injury/Plastic surgery

- Chest pain/Cardiac issues

# Chapter Eight:

# Staying Connected

One of the most difficult things about being in charge of your health is the ever changing information on almost everything that affects it. If you've experienced the 180 degree shifts on whether things like fats are bad or good you've felt the confusion along with the rest of us. You'll find riding the rollercoaster of changing recommendations is not easy. A good example of how "what's best" can change on a dime was the concern about fats in our foods. It was a major news event when it was announced that fats were causing an epidemic of obesity. This resulted in a flood of low-fat products on the market. The fats in the old products were replaced with sugars and it now appears that sugars are the devil behind much of the problem, along with their alter ego, artificial sweeteners. The final information on all things nutritional is still evolving. Researchers are finding exciting information every day. This is where each of us has to do our own due diligence.

You've certainly gotten the impression by now that the pages of this book are hoped to motivate, inspire and cheer you on to accomplish your health goals. It's such an important part of who you are and how you enjoy life. It's equally important that you're the person in charge, as only you know exactly how you feel about everything concerning you!

To help you connect to what's new you can visit NoOneShouldCareMoreAboutYourHealthThanYou.com, where you'll find information on everything from healthy food swaps to recipes and even the latest guru on the health scene! You'll be able to tap into articles and videos that will motivate you and help you keep focused and most of all interested in all that's healthy!

You'll find the Health Tip in A Minute newsletter at:

www.NewEnglandIntegrativeHealthCoach.com

# Some of my Favorite Things

90 for Life Vitamin Mineral Supplement: (Ultimate Tangy Tangerine)
http://changingthewayyoushop.com/


Life Spa Oral & Respiratory Defense & Flora Restore Max

http://tinyurl.com/p77rhr8


Canus Goat Milk Soap

http://www.canusgoatsmilk.com


Dr. Weil makes Tuscan Kale Salad

http://tinyurl.com/7bd3x82


Health Ranger Select Lavender Deodorant

http://tinyurl.com/qdp3wor


AMASAI Raspberry:  http://tinyurl.com/osu53q2

Mo Green Juice:  http://www.mogreenjuice.com/

Clean Plates Restaurant Guide:
http://www.cleanplates.com/

Omega 3  Moxxor:
http://integrativehealth.moxxor.com/

If you have a passion for health and wellness,
check in here about the coolest job in health!
http://geti.in/1D4MIIv

# Epilog:

# The power of synchronicity

I won't be able to do justice in just one chapter to the total effects that synchronicity has played in my life. So many times I've had crazy things pop up that move me to take a different path than the one I was on. The only recommendation I can make is that you really have to be looking at all times for subtle pulls that draw you.

Many such synchronicities happened during my husband's hospital stay. I, the caregiver and chief dog attender, was pretty tired as the journey went on. One of the days my day started with five one-hour calls with health coach students. I really wondered how I could focus for all five calls.

The order of the day was to first coach and then hurry to the hospital. To keep sane on the way I headed to a great local café called The Brown Cow. The Brown Cow Café has the best Chai Lattes and healthy whole foods! Then, of course, a swing by Dunkin Donuts for the patient's regular coffee. (Now I've told you our guilty vices!) That day I arrived just in time to run into one of the surgeons who had been involved while my husband's doctor was away. It was good timing to see him and be able to thank him for his care. Later that same day I ran into another covering surgeon, who by the way had gone out of his way to come back to the hospital late in the evening when needed. It's funny how you run with an urge that it's time to stretch your legs or run to grab a tea and then it unfolds why you were urged into action. A little later that day I ran downstairs to the hospital café and there was the receptionist who had started the ball rolling in the beginning of this saga, getting the initial appointment just in the nick of time. Another hug and another opportunity to say thank you and let her know how important she is! I was in the right place at the right time all day! (How are you at listening to the messages life's sending you? Do you fight against them or follow along?)


Here's my favorite example of synchronicity during that stressful time. It points out that when you pay attention to those unexpected cues they can urge you to remain calm even when you meet with annoying delays. It points out how it's good to wait it out. Often you'll see WHY things happen the way they do.

It was finally going-home day and I was

hustling to get to the hospital before the surgeon's morning visit. I was way ahead of schedule but on the way I received a call from my husband. He said that the doctor had already been there. BUMMER!! I had stopped to get coffee and a green tea (skipping that extra stop at the Brown Cow Café.) but I still wasn't early enough. I was fussing over missing the doctor's visit on such an important day (with all my so well-thought-out questions now unanswered). Unfortunately I was only given part of my order, the tea, and then I had to make an extra effort and spend more time to go back and retrieve the patient's coffee, the one thing I didn't want to leave without! It was a day of roadblocks in my path and I wasn't making very good time. But I'd missed his surgeon so, although I was upset about that, I no longer needed to hurry. Finally at the hospital, I didn't walk my usual long way around which I'd do to try to get some exercise. Many of you can relate that hospital visits are long days of sitting. At the spot where I usually passed by the elevators to the upper floor, that day I just pushed for the elevator to take that unusual alternate route. I remember thinking to myself as I got in "I don't like taking these elevators." Upstairs as I rounded the corner I almost ran right into my husband's doctor. Although startled, I remembered to ask the questions I had prepared and I got the full story of what was next. Even as we were talking I was running the scenario in my head of what it would have looked like if I had taken my normal route, with the two of us passing each other one above the other on different floors! That particular day I was so happy I had gone the way the day had pulled.

As it turned out my husband was going HOME! And I was able to feel secure that I'd asked the questions I needed to ask. Try going with your urges and watching what develops.

www.ingramcontent.com/pod-product-compliance
Lightning Source LLC
Chambersburg PA
CBHW070551290526
45790CB00002B/643